Mediterranean

A Definitive Guide Lower Your Blood Pressure And Improve Your Health

Written By

HOLLIE MCCARTHY, RDN

Table of Contents

INTRODUCTION

Thank you for purchasing this book!

The Mediterranean diet **protects against the onset of many types of cancer, including breast, colorectal, prostate, stomach, and liver**. The merit is **the richness of antioxidants, which counteract cell degeneration caused by free radicals, and the low content of fats (mostly unsaturated, such as beneficial omega-3 anti-inflammatory action).** To this is added the high content of fibers, which improving the intestinal transit make sure that potentially dangerous substances do not stay too long in contact with the walls of the intestine (a risk factor for colorectal cancer). **There are also substances with specific anti-tumor action present in some vegetables. Among these, glucosinolates of cruciferous vegetables (broccoli, cauliflower) and sulfur compounds in which onions are rich.**

Enjoy your reading!

BREAKFAST

Bacon, red pepper, and mozzarella frittata

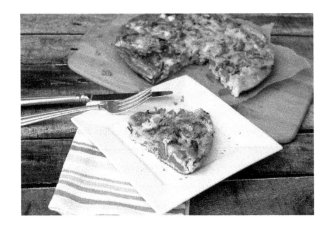

SERVES: 2

INGREDIENTS

- 7 slices Bacon
- 1 tbsp. Olive Oil
- 4 large Bella Mushroom Caps
- 2 tbsp. Fresh Parsley (Garnish)
- 1/2 Cup Chopped Fresh Basil
- 4 oz. Fresh Mozzarella Cheese, Cubed
- 2 oz. Goat Cheese, Grated
- 1 medium Red Bell Pepper
- 8-9 large Eggs
- 1/4 cup Heavy Cream
- 1/4 cup Parmesan Cheese, Grated
- Salt and Pepper to taste

DIRECTIONS

1. Preheat oven to 350F. Prep all of your vegetables first. Roughly chop 1 medium Red Bell Pepper, 7 Slices of Bacon, enough basil to turn into 1/2 cup, and 4 large Baby Bella Mushroom caps (remove stems before chopping).

2. In a hot pan, add 1 tbsp. olive oil. When the first wisp of smoke appears, add bacon to the pan immediately.

3. Cook the bacon just enough so that it starts to turn brown. Once that happens, add the chopped red bell pepper. Stir well.

4. While the red pepper is cooking, prep the egg mixture. Add 8 or 9 large eggs to a large mixing bowl along with 1/4 cup heavy cream, 1/4 cup parmesan cheese, and freshly ground pepper. Remember that parmesan has a salty quality to it so you shouldn't need to add extra salt here.

5. Using a whisk, whisk the egg mixture well so that everything is combined.

6. Once your red bell peppers begin to soften, add mushrooms to the pan and stir in well. You want the mushrooms to begin soaking up all the extra fats in the pan.

7. While the mushrooms are soaking up the fats, chop your 4 oz. fresh mozzarella into cubes.

8. Add the basil to the top of your ingredients and let it steam for a moment.

9. Sprinkle the mozzarella cubes on top of all the bacon and veggies.

10. Add your egg mixture to the pan, making sure it's evenly distributed.

11. 1Using your spoon, slowly mix the ingredients and "lift" the ingredients up so that the egg can get to the bottom of the pan. You want the eggs to be all around and underneath the bacon, red pepper, and mushrooms.

12. 1Grate 2 oz. of goat cheese over the top of the frittata, then put it in the oven for about 6-8 minutes at 350F. Leave the frittata in the pan and turn the broiler on. Broil for an additional 4-6 minutes, or until the top is started to turn golden brown.

13. 1Remove the frittata from the oven and let rest for 30-45 seconds.

14. 1Using a spoon, pry the edges of the frittata away from the pan. Make sure that all of the sides are easy to come off.

15. 1Flip the frittata out of the pan by placing a baking sheet with parchment paper over the top of it.

16. 1Once out of the pan, use a cutting board to flip the frittata right side up.

17. Garnish with 2 tbsp. fresh chopped parsley and slice!

NUTRITIONAL VALUES

408 Calories, 32g Fats, 4g Net Carbs, and 12g Protein.

Ultimate coffee cake

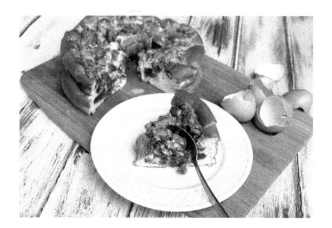

SERVES: 8

INGREDIENTS

Base

- 6 Large Eggs, Separated
- 6 Oz. Cream Cheese
- 1/4 cup Erythritol
- 1/4 tsp. Liquid Stevia
- 1/4 Cup Unflavored Protein Powder
- 2 tsp. Vanilla Extract
- 1/4 tsp. Cream of Tartar

Filling

- 1 1/2 Cup Almond Flour
- 1 Tbsp. Cinnamon
- 1/2 Stick Butter

- 1/4 cup Maple Syrup
- 1/4 cup Erythritol

DIRECTIONS

1. Preheat your oven to 325F. If you're using a glass baking dish, use 300F.
2. Separate the eggs from the egg whites for all 5 eggs. Cream together the egg yolks with 1/4 cup Erythritol and 1/4 tsp. Liquid Stevia.
3. Once the egg yolks are creamed, add 6 Oz. Cream cheese and 1/4 Cup Un-
4. flavored Protein Powder. Mix this well until a thick batter forms.
5. Beat your egg whites together with the 1/4 tsp. Cream of Tartar until stiff peaks form.
6. Fold the egg whites into the egg yolk mixture, doing 1/2 of the egg whites first and then the other half. Pour the batter into a round cake pan.
7. Mix all of the "Filling" ingredients: 1 1/2 Cup Almond Flour, 1
8. Tbsp. Cinnamon, 1/2 Stick Butter, 1/4 Cup Maple Syrup, and ¼ Cup Erythritol. This should form a "dough" of sorts. Take half and rip off little pieces to top the cake – push the pieces down if they don't sink on their own.
9. Bake for 20 minutes and then top with the rest of the cinnamon filling. Bake for another 20-30 minutes until a toothpick comes out clean. Let cool for 20 minutes before removing from the cake pan.

NUTRITIONAL VALUES

257 Calories, 27g Fats, 8g Net Carbs, and 18g Protein.

Peanut butter pancakes

- **SERVES: 2**
-
- **INGREDIENTS**
- 4 Tbsp. Heavy Cream
- 4 Tbsp. Golden Flaxseed
- 2 Large Eggs
- 2 Tbsp. Peanut Butter
- 2 Tbsp. Maple Syrup
- 1/2 tsp. Baking Powder
- 1 Tbsp. Butter(Grease the Pan)

DIRECTIONS

1. Mix 2 Tbsp. Peanut Butter, 2 Tbsp. Maple Syrup and 2large eggs.
2. Once the peanut butter is starting to break up, add the 4 Tbsp. Heavy Cream.
3. Mix once more and then add the 4 Tbsp. Golden Flaxseed and 1/2 tsp. Baking Powder. Mix everything well until a pancake batter has formed.
4. Grease a pan with a little bit of butter under medium-low heat. Once the pan is hot, you can add your pancake batter to form whichever size pancakes you'd like. You can get an awesome ring mold to help with cooking

5. Cook the pancakes until the sides are starting to harden up and the top is bubbling. Remove your ring mold from the pancake and it should stand by itself. Once it is like this, use a spatula to flip the pancake over. Cook for an additional 1-2 minutes.

6. Set aside pancakes and cook more as needed. Top with butter and maple syrup if you'd like!

This yields 2 servings.

NUTRITIONAL VALUES

389 Calories, 39g Fats, 8g Net Carbs, and 15g Protein.

Garden Scramble (Vegan)

SERVES: 4

INGREDIENTS

- 1 pound firm tofu, drained, crumbled, and squeezed dry
- ¼ cup nutritional yeast
- 1 teaspoon onion powder
- ½ teaspoon garlic powder
- ½ teaspoon ground cumin
- ¼ teaspoon turmeric
- ½ teaspoon salt
- ¼ teaspoon freshly ground black pepper
- 1 tablespoon olive oil
- 1 small red onion, minced
- ½ cup minced red bell pepper
- cremini mushrooms, lightly rinsed, patted dry, and thinly sliced
- 1 medium carrot, shredded
- 1 tablespoon soy sauce
- 1 cup fresh or thawed frozen peas
- cilantro or parsley sprigs, for garnish

DIRECTIONS

1. In a large bowl, combine the tofu, nutritional yeast, and dry spices and mix well. Set aside.

2. In a large skillet, heat the oil over medium heat. Add the onion, cover, and cook until tender, about 5 minutes. Add the bell pepper, mushrooms, and carrot and cook uncovered about 5 minutes longer. Stir in the soy sauce.

3. Add the tofu mixture and stir until hot and well combined. Add the peas and stir to combine. Cook, stirring the mixture until it is hot and any excess moisture has evaporated about 5 minutes.

4. Serve hot or warm plates and garnish with sprigs of cilantro.

LUNCH

Southwestern pork stew

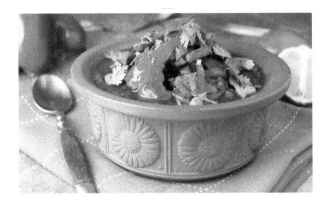

SERVES: 4

INGREDIENTS

- 1 lb. Cooked Pork Shoulder, sliced
- 2 tsp. Chili Powder
- 2 tsp. Cumin
- 1 tsp. Minced Garlic
- 1/2 tsp. Salt
- 1/2 tsp. Pepper
- 1 tsp. Paprika
- 1 tsp. Oregano
- 1/4 tsp. Cinnamon
- 2 Bay Leafs
- 6 oz. Button Mushrooms
- 1/2 sliced Jalapeno
- 1/2 medium Onion

- 1/2 Green Bell Pepper, sliced
- 1/2 Red Bell Pepper, sliced
- Juice 1/2 Lime (to finish)
- 2 cups Gelatinous Bone Broth
- 2 cup Chicken Broth
- 1/2 cup Strong Coffee
- 1/4 cup Tomato Paste

DIRECTIONS

1. Prep all vegetables by slicing and chopping them.
2. Let your bone broth start to come to room temperature. This is my bone broth that I made with the pork bones – I will post a recipe on this sometime in the future.
3. Bring a pan to high heat with 2 tbsp. Olive Oil. Once hot, add vegetables and sauté them until they are slightly cooked and aromatic.
4. Measure out all spices into a small container so you can use them as needed.
5. Slice pork (I use the tougher meat for this) into bite-size chunks.
6. Add bone broth, chicken broth, and coffee to the slow cooker.
7. Add pork and mushrooms to the slow cooker and mix.
8. Add spices and vegetables (with oil) to the slow cooker. Mix well, cover, and set on low for 4-10 hours.
9. Once it's finished, take the lid off and stir together.
10. Serve it up!

NUTRITIONAL VALUES

386 Calories, 29g Fats, 4g Net Carbs, and 19g Protein.

Thai bbq pork salad

SERVES: 2

INGREDIENTS

The Salad

- 10 oz. Pulled Pork
- 2 cups Romaine Lettuce
- 1/4 cup Cilantro, chopped
- 1/4 medium Red Bell Pepper, Chopped

The Sauce

- 2 tbsp. Tomato Paste
- 2 tbsp. + 2 tsp. Soy Sauce (or coconut)
- 1 tbsp. Creamy Peanut Butter
- 2 tbsp. Cilantro, chopped
- Juice & Zest of 1/2 Lime
- 1 tsp. Five Spice
- 1 tsp. Red Curry Paste
- 1 tbsp. + 1 tsp. Rice Wine Vinegar
- 1/4 tsp. Red Pepper Flakes
- 1 tsp. Fish Sauce
- 10 drops Liquid Stevia
- 1/2 tsp. Mango Extract

DIRECTIONS

1. In a bowl, combine all the sauce ingredients (except for cilantro and lime zest).
2. Chop cilantro and zest a lime and add to the sauce.
3. Mix the Thai BBQ sauce well, and then set aside.
4. Using your fingers, or a knife, pull apart the pork.
5. That's it! Assemble the salad and glaze over the pork with some sauce.
6. Depending on how you like it, you may have extra sauce to work with so you can save it for another salad!

NUTRITIONAL VALUES

461 Calories, 36g Fats, 2g Net Carbs, and 22g Protein.

DINNER

Low-carb chicken curry

SERVES: 3

INGREDIENTS

- 2 tbsp. Coconut Oil
- 5 inch Ginger
- 1 medium Green Chilli
- 2 small Shallots
- 2 cloves Garlic
- 2 tsp. Turmeric Powder
- 1 stalk Lemongrass
- 1/2 cup Coconut Milk
- 1/2 cup Water
- 6 small Chicken Drumsticks (~21 oz. bone-in)
- 1/2 tsp. Salt
- 1 tbsp. Cilantro, chopped
-

DIRECTIONS

1   Bruise 1 stalk Lemongrass. This will help release the aroma when cooking.
2   With a pestle and mortar, pound 5 inch Ginger, 1 Green Chili, 2 Shallots, and 2 cloves Garlic. Alternatively, you can use a blender.
3   In a pre-heated pot over medium heat, melt 2 tbsp. Coconut Oil. Once hot, add in the pounded ingredients and sauté.

4   After 3-4 minutes, add in 2 tsp. Turmeric Powder and the smashed Lemongrass and sauté once again.

5   Add in chicken meat and mix well with the sautéed ingredients.

6   Once the meat is coated, pour in 1/2 cup each Coconut Milk and Water.

7   Add in 1/2 tsp. Salt and cover the pot. Let everything cook for about 20 minutes or until desired thickness is reached and chicken is cooked through.

8   Sprinkle 1 tbsp. chopped cilantro over the top and serve!

NUTRITIONAL VALUES

493 Calories, 35g Protein, 8g Net Carbs, and 35g Protein.

Thai chicken zoodles

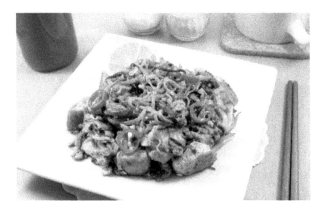

SERVES: 1

INGREDIENTS

- 1/2 tsp. Curry Powder
- 5 oz. Chicken Thigh
- 1 tbsp. Unsalted Butter
- 1 tbsp. Coconut Oil
- 1 stalk Spring Onion
- 1 clove Garlic
- 1 large Egg
- 4 oz. Bean Sprouts
- 5 oz. Zucchini
- 1 tsp. Soy Sauce
- 1/2 tsp. Oyster Sauce
- 1/8 tsp. White Pepper
- 1 tsp. Lime Juice

- Red Chilies, chopped
- Salt and Pepper to Taste

DIRECTIONS

1 Season the chicken with 1/2 tsp. Curry Powder and a pinch of Salt and Pepper. Keep aside for a while.

2 Prepare the sauce by combining 1 tsp. Soy Sauce, 1/2 tsp. Oyster Sauce, and 1/8 tsp. White Pepper.

3 Finely chop Spring Onion and Garlic and make Zoodles out of Zucchini. I use this spiralizer to do so.

4 Fry the seasoned Chicken with 1 tbsp. Unsalted Butter until brown. When done, slice to bite-sized pieces.

5 In the same pan, melt 1 tbsp. Coconut Oil on high heat. Sauté chopped Spring Onion until fragrant.

6 Add chopped Garlic and again sauté until fragrant.

7 Crack an egg into the pan and make a scrambled egg. Sauté until slightly brown.

8 Add in Bean Sprouts and Zoodles. Mix everything well together.

9 Add in the sauce and stir. Reduce until there is little liquid left.

10 Add in the fried chicken pieces and stir.

11 Garnish with a few chopped Red Chilies and squeeze some Lime Juice on top. Serve while

NUTRITIONAL VALUES

580 Calories, 41g Fats, 8g Net Carbs, and 28g Protein.

SNACKS

Chocolate chunk cookies

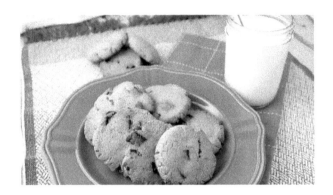

SERVES: 4

INGREDIENTS

- 1 cup Almond Flour
- 3 tbsp. Unflavored Whey Protein
- 2 tbsp. Coconut Flour
- 2 tbsp. Psyllium Husk Pow
- tbsp. Unsalted Butter
- 2 tsp. Quality Vanilla Extract
- 1/4 cup Erythritol
- drops Liquid Stevia
- 1/2 tsp. Baking Powder
- 1 large Egg
- bars Choco perfection

DIRECTIONS

1. Preheat the oven to 350F. Then, mix 1 cup Almond Flour, 3 tbsp. Unflavored Whey Protein, 2 tbsp. Coconut Flour, 2 tbsp. Psyllium Husk Powder and 1/2 tsp. Baking Powder.
2. Using a hand mixer, beat 8 tbsp. room temperature butter to a pale color.
3. Add 1/4 cup Erythritol and 10 drops Liquid Stevia to the butter and beat again.
4. Add 1 large egg and 2 tsp. Quality Vanilla Extract to the beaten butter and beat again until well combined.
5. Sift dry ingredients over butter and mix again to combine fully. Make sure there are no lumps when you finish.
6. Chop the 5 bars of Chocoperfection (or other 95%+ Cocoa) and add to the dough. Mix well.
7. Roll the dough into a log. Make small markings over the top of the log to ensure consistent measurements of cookies.
8. Slice off each piece of dough and roll into a ball. Lay each ball onto a pat that is on a baking sheet.
9. Using the bottom of a mason jar, lightly press the cookies flat into circles.
10. Bake the cookies for 12-15 minutes or until a light golden brown color appears on the edges.
11. Let cool for 5-10 minutes before removing from the baking sheet.
12. Serve up with a nice glass of coconut or almond milk, and enjoy!

This Makes 16 total Chocolate Chunk Cookies.

NUTRITIONAL VALUES

Each cookie will have 118 Calories, 8g Fats, 6g Net Carbs, and 6g Protein.

Goat cheese tomato tarts

SERVES: 6 yo 12

INGREDIENTS

Roasted Tomatoes

- 2 medium Tomatoes, Cut into 1/4 Slices
- 1/4 cup Olive Oil
- Salt & Pepper to Taste

Tart Base

- 1/2 cup Almond Flour
- 1 tbsp. Psyllium Husk
- 2 tbsp. Coconut Flour
- tbsp. Cold Butter, Cubed
- 1/4 tsp. Salt

Tart Filling

- 1/2 medium Onion, Sliced Thin
- 3 oz. Goat Cheese
- 2 tbsp. Olive Oil
- 2 tsp. Minced Garlic
- 3 tsp. fresh Thyme

DIRECTIONS

1. Preheat oven to 425F, then slice 2 medium tomatoes into 1/4 slices. You should get at least 6 slices per tomato.
2. Lay slices on a baking sheet with parchment paper, then drizzle with 1/4 cup olive oil and season with salt and pepper to taste.
3. Bake the tomatoes for 30-40 minutes or until they are roasted and have lost most of their juice.
4. Set the tomatoes aside.
5. In a food processor, combine 1/2 cup Almond Flour, 1 tbsp. Psyllium Husk, 2 tbsp. Coconut Flour, and 1/4 tsp. Salt.
6. Cube 5 tbsp. Cold Butter and add it to the food processor also.
7. Slowly pulse the ingredients until the dough starts to form.
8. Press dough into silicone cupcake molds. You want to make sure these layers are quite thin. About 1/4 – 1/2 thick.
9. Reduce oven heat to 350F and bake the tarts at 350F for 17-20 minutes or until golden brown.
10. Remove tarts from the oven and let cool. Once cooled, turn the silicone cupcake molds upside down and lightly tap the bottom so that the tart dough falls out.
11. 1Layer tomato onto each tart and set aside for a moment.
12. 1Slice 1/2 medium onion thin, then caramelize the onion and 2 tsp. minced garlic in 2 tbsp. olive oil.
13. 1Add caramelized onions and garlic on top of the tomato.
14. 1Crumble goat cheese and sprinkle fresh thyme over each tart, then bake for an additional 5-6 minutes or until the cheese begins to melt.
15. 1Serve warm!

NUTRITIONAL VALUES

Each tart will have 162 Calories, 16g Fats, 1g Net Carbs, and 8g Protein.

SIDE DISHES

Asian cucumber salad

SERVES: 2

INGREDIENTS

- 3/4 large Cucumber
- 1 packet Shirataki Noodles
- 2 tbsp. Coconut Oil
- 1 medium Spring Onion
- 1/4 tsp. Red Pepper Flakes
- 1 tbsp. Sesame Oil
- 1 tbsp. Rice Vinegar
- 1 tsp. Sesame Seeds
- Salt and Pepper to Taste

DIRECTIONS

1. Remove shiritaki noodles from the package and rise off completely. This may take a few minutes, but make sure that all of the extra water that came in its package is washed off.
2. Set noodles on a kitchen towel and thoroughly dry them.
3. Bring 2 tbsp. Coconut Oil to medium-high heat in a pan.
4. Once the oil is hot, add noodles and cover (it will splatter). Let these fry for 5-7 minutes or until crisp and browned.
5. Remove shiritaki noodles from the pan and set on paper towels to cool and dry.
6. Slice cucumber thin and arrange on a plate in the design you'd like.

7 Add 1 medium Spring Onion, 1/4 tsp. Red Pepper Flakes, 1 tbsp. Sesame Oil, 1 tbsp. Rice Vinegar, 1 tsp. Sesame Seeds, and Salt and Pepper to taste. You can also pour over the coconut oil from the pan you fried the noodles in.

8 This will add a salty component so keep that in mind. Store this in the fridge for at least 30 minutes before serving!

Low carb flax tortillas

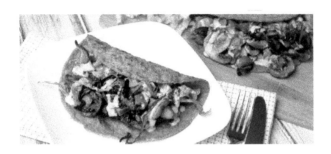

SERVES: 5

INGREDIENTS

- 1 cup Golden Flax Seed Meal
- 2 tbsp. Psyllium Husk Powder
- 2 tsp. Olive Oil
- 1/4 tsp. Xanthan Gum
- 1/2 tsp. Curry Powder (or spices of your choice)
- 1 cup + 2 tbsp. Filtered Water

DIRECTIONS

1   Add 1 cup Golden Flax Seed Meal, 2 tbsp. Psyllium Husk Powder, 1/4 tsp. Xanthan Gum, and 1/2 tsp. Curry Powder (or spices of your choice) in a mixing bowl.

2   Mix the entire dry ingredients well, making sure all of the powders are evenly distributed.

3   Add 2 tsp. Olive Oil and 1 cup + 2 tbsp. Filtered Water to the mixture. Mix this well until a solid ball forms out of the mixture.

4   Leave this uncovered for 1 hour on the countertop

5   With each portion, press it against the Silpat using your hand.

6   Sprinkle ~1/2 tsp. coconut flour over the tortilla and rolling pin, roll out the dough as thin as you can get it without tearing it.

7   Using a large round object, for me, it was the lid of a pan, cut out your tortilla and separate it from the excess dough. Take the excess dough and save it to roll out more tortillas.

8   You should be left with a completely round tortilla. Repeat the process for each tortilla.

9   In a pan over medium-high heat, add 1 tsp. olive oil.

10 Once the oil is hot, add tortilla and fry to browning of your choosing.

11 OPTIONAL (But really, when is frying bacon optional?): Fry up some bacon.

12 OPTIONAL: Add mushrooms, green pepper, and red cabbage to bacon fat and let it soak up all the fats.

13 Serve! Feel free to add fillings of your choice!

This makes 5 total Flax Tortillas.

NUTRITIONAL VALUES

Each tortilla has 165 Calories, 14g Fats, 0.5g Net Carbs, and 6g Protein

DESSERT

No-Bake Fresh Fruit Pie

SERVES: 8

INGREDIENTS

- 1½ cups vegan oatmeal cookie crumbs
- ¼ cup vegan margarine
- 1 pound firm tofu, well-drained and pressed (see Tofu)
- ¾ cup sugar
- 1 teaspoon pure vanilla extract
- 1 ripe peach, pitted and cut into ¼-inch slices
- 2 ripe plums, pitted and cut into ¼-inch slices
- ¼ cup peach preserves
- 1 teaspoon fresh lemon juice

DIRECTIONS

1   Grease a 9-inch pie plate and set it aside. In a food processor, combine the crumbs and the melted margarine and process until the crumbs are moistened. Press the crumb mixture into the prepared pie plate. Refrigerate until needed.

2   In the food processor, combine the tofu, sugar, and vanilla and process until smooth. Spread the tofu mixture into the chilled crust and refrigerate for 1 hour.

3   Arrange the fruit decoratively on top of the tofu mixture. Set aside.

4   In a small heatproof bowl, combine the preserves and lemon juice and microwave until melted, about 5 seconds. Stir and drizzle over the fruit. Refrigerate the pie for at least 1 hour before serving to chill the filling and set the glaze.

Cashew–Banana Cream Pie

SERVES: 8

DIRECTIONS

- 1½ cups vegan vanilla cookie crumbs
- ¼ cup vegan margarine, melted
- ½ cup unsalted raw cashews
- 1 (13-ounce) can unsweetened coconut milk
- ⅔ cup sugar
- ripe bananas
- 1 tablespoon agar flakes
- 1 teaspoon pure vanilla extract
- 1 teaspoon coconut extract (optional)
- Vegan Whipped Cream, homemade or store-bought, and toasted coconut, for garnish

DIRECTIONS

1   Lightly oil the bottom and sides of an 8-inch springform pan or pie plate and set aside. In a food processor, combine the cookie crumbs and margarine and pulse until the crumbs are moistened. Press the crumb mixture into the bottom and sides of the prepared pan. Refrigerate until needed.

2 In a high-speed blender, grind the cashews to a powder. Add the coconut milk, sugar, and one of the bananas and blend until smooth. Scrape the mixture into a saucepan, add the agar flakes, and set aside for 10 minutes to soften the agar. Bring just to a boil, then reduce the heat to low and simmer, stirring constantly to dissolve the agar, about 3 minutes. Remove from the heat and stir in the lemon juice, vanilla, and coconut extract, if using. Set aside.

3 Cut the remaining 2 bananas into $\frac{1}{4}$-inch slices and arrange evenly in the bottom of the prepared

4 pan. Spread the cashew-banana mixture into the pan, then refrigerate until well chilled. When ready to serve, garnish with whipped cream and toasted coconut. Store leftovers covered in the refrigerator.

Peanut Butter–Ice Cream Pie

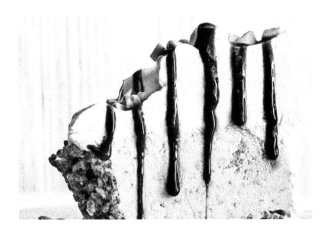

SERVES: 8

INGREDIENTS

- 1½ cups vegan chocolate cookie crumbs
- ¼ cup vegan margarine, melted
- 1-quart vegan vanilla ice cream softened
- 2 cups creamy peanut butter
- Vegan chocolate curls, for garnish

DIRECTIONS

1   Lightly oil the bottom and sides of a 9-inch springform pan and set it aside. In a food processor, combine the cookie crumbs and margarine and process until the crumbs are moistened. Press the crumb mixture into the prepared pan and press into the bottom and sides of the pan. Refrigerate until needed.

2   In a food processor, combine the ice cream and peanut butter, mixing until well blended. Spread the mixture evenly into the prepared crust.

3   Freeze for 3 hours or overnight. Bring the pie to room temperature for 5 minutes and carefully remove the sides of the springform pan. Sprinkle chocolate curls over the top of the pie and serve.

Banana Mango Pie

SERVES: 6

INGREDIENTS

- 1½ cups vegan vanilla cookie crumbs
- ¼ cup vegan margarine, melted
- 1 cup mango juice
- 1 tablespoon agar flakes
- ¼ cup agave nectar
- ripe bananas, peeled and cut into chunks
- 1 teaspoon fresh lemon juice
- 1 fresh ripe mango, peeled, pitted, and thinly sliced

DIRECTIONS

1   Grease the bottom and sides of an 8-inch pie plate. Place the cookie crumbs and the melted margarine in the bottom of the pie plate and stir with a fork to combine until the crumbs are moistened. Press into the bottom and sides of the prepared pie plate. Refrigerate until needed.

2   Combine the juice and agar flakes in a small saucepan. Let it sit for 10 minutes to soften. Add the agave nectar and bring the mixture just to a boil. Reduce the heat to a simmer and stir until dissolved, about 3 minutes.

3   Place the bananas in a food processor and process until smooth. Add the agar mixture and lemon juice and process until smooth and well blended. Use a rubber spatula to scrape the filling into the prepared crust. Refrigerate for 2 hours or longer to chill and set up.

4   Just before serving, arrange the mango slices in a circle on top of the pie.

Two-Berry Cobbler

SERVES: 8

INGREDIENTS

- 2 cups blueberries
- ¾ cup sugar
- 1 tablespoon cornstarch
- ¼ cup water
- 1 cup canned whole-berry cranberry sauce
- 1½ cups all-purpose flour
- ½ teaspoon ground cinnamon
- 2 teaspoons baking powder
- ½ teaspoon salt
- ⅓ cup vegan margarine, melted
- ½ cup plain or vanilla soy milk

DIRECTIONS

1   Preheat the oven to 375°F. In a saucepan, combine the blueberries, ½ cup of the sugar, cornstarch,

2   water, and cinnamon, stirring to blend. Bring to a boil over high heat, then reduce heat to low, and stir gently until slightly thickened about 5 minutes.

3   Remove the saucepan from the heat and stir in the cranberry sauce until well mixed. Spoon the fruit mixture into the bottom of a 9-inch square baking pan and set aside.

4   In a large bowl, combine the flour, baking powder, salt, and remaining ¼ cup sugar. Blend in the margarine and soy milk until a soft dough forms. Drop the dough by large spoonfuls on top of the fruit mixture. Bake until the fruit is bubbly and the top of the crust is golden brown, about 40 minutes. Serve warm.

Apple And Pear Cobbler

SERVES: 6

INGREDIENTS

- Granny Smith apples, peeled, cored, and shredded
- 2 ripe pears, peeled, cored, and cut into ¼-inch slices
- 2 teaspoons fresh lemon juice
- ½ cup plus 2 tablespoons sugar
- 2 tablespoons cornstarch
- 1 teaspoon ground cinnamon
- ½ teaspoon ground allspice
- 1 cup all-purpose flour
- 1½ teaspoons baking powder
- ¼ teaspoon salt
- 2 tablespoons canola or other neutral oil
- ½ cup plain or vanilla soy milk

DIRECTIONS

1. Preheat the oven to 400°F.
2. Grease a 9-inch square baking pan.
3. Spread the apples and pears in the prepared pan. Sprinkle with the lemon juice and toss to coat. Stir in ½ cup of the sugar, cornstarch, cinnamon, and allspice, stirring to mix.
4. In a medium bowl, combine the flour, the remaining 2 tablespoons sugar, the baking powder, and the salt.

5. Add the oil and mix with a fork until the mixture resembles coarse crumbs.

6. Mix in the soy milk.

7. Spread the topping over the fruit. Bake until golden, about 30 minutes. Serve warm.

Blueberry-Peach Crisp

SERVES: 8

INGREDIENTS

- fresh ripe peaches, peeled, pitted, and cut into ¼-inch slices
- 2 cups fresh blueberries
- 1 tablespoon cornstarch
- ¾ cup sugar
- 2 teaspoons fresh lemon juice
- 1 teaspoon ground cinnamon
- ½ cup all-purpose flour
- ½ cup old-fashioned oats
- 2 tablespoons vegan margarine

DIRECTIONS

1. Preheat the oven to 375°F. Lightly oil a 9-inch square baking pan and set it aside.
2. In a large bowl, combine the peaches, blueberries, cornstarch, ¼ cup of the sugar, lemon juice, and ½ teaspoon of the cinnamon.
3. Mix gently and spoon into the prepared baking pan. Set aside.
4. In a small bowl, combine the flour, oats, margarine, the remaining ½ cup sugar, and the remaining ½ teaspoon cinnamon. Use a pastry blender or fork to mix until crumbly.
5. Sprinkle the topping over the fruit mixture and bake until the top is browned and bubbly in the center, 30 to 40 minutes. Serve warm.

Quick Apple Crisp

SERVES: 6

INGREDIENTS

- Granny Smith apples, peeled, cored, and cut into ¼-inch slices
- 1 tablespoon fresh lemon juice
- 1 teaspoon ground cinnamon
- ½ cup all-purpose flour
- ½ cup old-fashioned oats
- ½ cup finely chopped walnuts or pecans
- ⅔ cup light brown sugar
- ½ cup vegan margarine, softened

DIRECTIONS

1. Preheat the oven to 350°F. Lightly oil a 9-inch square baking pan.
2. Place the apples in the prepared pan. Drizzle the maple syrup and lemon juice over the apples and sprinkle with ½ teaspoon of the cinnamon. Set aside.
3. In a medium bowl, mix the flour, oats, walnuts, sugar, and the remaining ½ teaspoon cinnamon.
4. Use a pastry blender to cut in the margarine until the mixture resembles coarse crumbs. Spread the topping over the apples and bake until bubbly and lightly browned on top, about 45 minutes. Serve warm.

Banana-Pecan Strudel

SERVES: 6

INGREDIENTS

- 2 tablespoons vegan margarine
- ½ cup light brown sugar
- 1 cup chopped unsalted pecans
- ripe bananas, sliced
- 2 tablespoons rum or 1 teaspoon rum extract (optional)
- ½ teaspoon ground cinnamon
- 1 sheet frozen puff pastry, thawed
- Sugar, for rolling and dusting pastry

DIRECTIONS

1. In a large skillet, melt the margarine over medium heat. Add the brown sugar and stir to blend. Add the pecans and bananas and cook for 1 minute, stirring to coat. Add the rum, if using, and the cinnamon and stir to combine. Remove from heat and set aside to cool.

2. Roll out the puff pastry on a lightly sugared work surface to eliminate the creases in the pastry.

3. Spread the cooled banana mixture down the length of the pastry. Fold the sides of the pastry over the banana mixture and tuck in the ends, sealing the edges with your fingers.

4. Place the strudel on an ungreased baking sheet and cut a few diagonal slashes on top of the pastry with a sharp knife to allow steam to escape.

5. Sprinkle a little sugar on the top of the strudel and refrigerate for 15 minutes. Preheat the oven to 400°F.

6. Bake the strudel until golden brown, 35 to 40 minutes. Cool for 10 minutes. Use a serrated bread knife to cut into slices and serve.

Pear Crumble

SERVES: 6

INGREDIENTS

- ripe Bartlett pears, peeled, cored, and cut into ¼-inch slices
- 2 tablespoons cornstarch
- 1 teaspoon ground allspice
- ½ teaspoon ground ginger
- 1 cup all-purpose flour
- ½ cup old-fashioned oats
- 1 cup sugar
- ½ cup vegan margarine, cut into small pieces

DIRECTIONS

1. Preheat the oven to 375°F.
2. Place the pear slices in a 9-inch square baking pan and sprinkle with the sugar, the cornstarch, ½ teaspoon of the allspice, and the ginger.
3. In a medium bowl, combine the flour, oats, sugar, and remaining ½ teaspoon of allspice. Use a pastry blender or fork to cut in the margarine until the mixture resembles coarse crumbs.
4. Spread the topping over the pears and bake until browned and bubbly, about 40 minutes. Serve warm.

MEDITERRANEAN SEAFOOD

Salmon with Basil Cream Sauce

SERVES: 2

INGREDIENTS

- 2 lbs.   salmon fillets
- 1 1/2 T unsalted butter
- 3 shallots, peeled and minced
- 1 clove garlic, peeled and minced
- 1 1/2 cup chopped fresh basil
- 1/4 cup chopped fresh parsley
- 3/4 cup dry white wine
- 1/3 cup light cream
- 1T freshly squeezed lemon juice
- 1/4 t   freshly ground white pepper
- 1/4 t   salt, or to taste

DIRECTIONS

1   Cut the salmon into 6 equal serving pieces, wash and pat dry on paper towels. Melt the butter in a large skillet over medium-high heat. Sear the salmon on each side for about 2 to

2   minutes, keeping the center slightly rare since the fish will continue to cook after it is taken from the pan.

3   Remove the fish from the pan with a slotted spatula and keep warm. Reduce the heat to low and add the shallots and garlic to the pan. Sauté, stirring frequently, for 5 minutes.

4   Add the basil, parsley, wine, cream, lemon juice, pepper, and salt to the pan and cook over medium heat, stirring frequently, until the mixture is reduced by half. Taste for seasoning, adding pepper and salt as needed.

5   To serve, reheat the fish slightly in the sauce and then serve the sauce around the salmon fillets.

6   NOTE: The fish can be prepared up to three hours in advance. Reheat the fish in the sauce over low heat, uncovered, for 10 minutes.

Spicy Salmon and Eggplant

SERVES: 4

INGREDIENTS

- 3 fresh salmon steaks
- eggplant
- limes
- lemons
- 1/8 cup olive oil
- 1 tsp. Greek or Italian seasoning 1/8 tsp. hot red pepper flakes Fresh ground black pepper

DIRECTIONS

1 Remove stem and end of eggplant and slice on a diagonal, cutting slices approximately 1/4-inch thick.

2 Place salmon steaks and eggplant slices in a large, flat Tupperware container. Cut lemons and limes in half and remove the juice.

3 Pour the juice into a separate bowl. Stir in olive oil, seasoning, pepper flakes, and ground pepper. Pour over steaks and eggplant. Cover and marinate in the refrigerator for 1 to 1-1/2 hours. Turn steaks over and rearrange eggplant for even marinating, once during the process. Place steaks on a hot grill and cook on both sides until done. Add eggplant slices to grill when fish is half cooked. Grill eggplant slices on both sides. Remove.

4 Serve fish and vegetables with rice.

Citrus Salmon

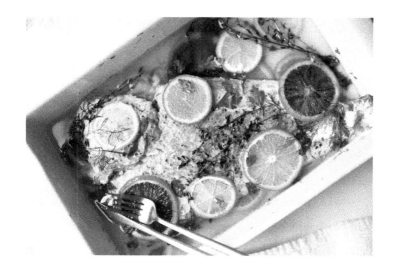

SERVES: 4

INGREDIENTS

- 1 lb (500g) salmon fillets
- Salt and pepper
- 1 tbsp   cornstarch
- 1 tbsp   water
- 2 tbsp   undiluted frozen orange juice concentrate
- 1 tbsp   lemon juice
- 1/4 cup brown sugar

Garnish (optional)

- 1 sliced orange
- parsley

DIRECTIONS

1   Sprinkle both sides of the salmon fillet with salt and pepper. Mix the corn-starch and water in a small bowl to form a paste. Add the orange juice concentrate, lemon juice, and brown sugar. Stir the mixture well until all the ingredients are dissolved. Set aside.

2   Pour half of the sauce into the bottom of a microwaveable dish. Place the salmon fillet in the dish on top of the sauce. Pour the remaining sauce over the salmon. Cover the dish with plastic wrap. Vent to allow steam to escape.

3   Microwave on high for 7-10 minutes (depending on microwave)

4   Remove from microwave and remove plastic wrap. Place the fillet on a plate.

5   Stir the remaining sauce and pour over the fillet and garnish if desired.

Thai salmon parcels

SERVES: 2

INGREDIENTS

2 4-5oz salmon fillets

4 sheets filo pastry

1 oz butter   zest & juice 1 lime

1 tsp grated ginger 1 clove garlic (pressed)

1 spring onion (finely chopped)

1 Tbsp fresh coriander (finely   chopped)

salt & pepper

DIRECTIONS

1   Mix lime zest and juice, garlic, spring onion, ginger, and coriander.

2   Melt butter. Lay out 1 sheet of filo, and brush with butter. Lay the second sheet on top, brush with more butter.

3   Lay a salmon fillet about 2-3 inches from the short side of the pastry, season to taste, and put half of the lime mixture on top.

4   Fold the short end of pastry over salmon, then fold in the 2 long sides. Fold the salmon over twice more, and cut off the remaining pastry. Do the same with the other fillet.

5   Put the parcels on a well-greased baking sheet, and just before a baking brush with the remaining butter. Cook at gas mark 5 for 20-25 Minutes, until brown and crispy.

Smoked Salmon Dip

SERVES: 4

INGREDIENTS

- Here's what you need:
- Light cream cheese-1 package (8 oz.)
- Lemon juice-3 Tbsp
- Low-fat milk-3 Tbsp
- Smoked Alaska salmon-1 package (8 to 12 oz.)
- Thinly sliced green onions-1/4 cup Crackers or
- French bread slices-as needed

DIRECTIONS

1 Mix cream cheese with lemon juice and milk until light and fluffy. Stir in salmon and green onions until thoroughly combined.

2 Put it together!

3 Spread on crackers or French bread slices.

4 Nutrients per serving: 386 calories, 16g total fat, 6g saturated fat, 144mg cholesterol, 51g protein, 7g carbohydrate, 2g fiber, 215mg sodium, 165mg calcium, and 2g omega-3 fatty acids.

Wild Salmon,Chive& Cheddar Grills

SERVES: 2

INGREDIENTS

- Canned sockeye (red) or 1tall(14.75oz.)
- pinkwild salmon-7.5 oz. cans
- Low-fat soft cheese with garlic and herbs-4 oz.
- Cheddar cheese, grated-2oz.
- Chopped chives-1 Tbsp
- Sourdough or mixed seed bread-4 thick slices

DIRECTIONS

1 Drain the canned salmon. Break the salmon into chunks.

2 Add the soft cheese and about two-thirds of the Cheddar to the salmon. Stir together with the chives.

3 Put it together!

4 Spread the salmon mixture over the slices of bread. Sprinkle the leftover Cheddar over the top, then place in the toaster oven until melted and bubbling. Serve at once.

5 Nutrients per serving: 453 calories, 19g total fat, 9g saturated fat, 108mg cholesterol, 38g protein, 30g carbohydrate, 1g fiber, 899mg sodium, 159mg calcium, and 1.5g omega-3 fatty acids.

Salmon Burgers

SERVES: 4

INGREDIENTS

- Canned sockeye (red) or pink salmon-1 tall (14.75 oz.) or 2 short (7.5 oz.) cans
- Egg-1 large
- Onion, diced (cut into small pieces)-1/2 cup
- Salt and pepper to taste
- Bread crumbs or crushed crackers-1/2 cup

DIRECTIONS

1   Drain salmon thoroughly. In a bowl, flake salmon with a fork. Add egg, onion, salt and pepper, and bread crumbs. Blend thoroughly until the mixture is almost smooth.
2   Divide equally and form mixture into four patties.
3   Preheat broiler/oven or grill to medium-high heat. Place patties on a spray-coated broiling pan or well-oiled grill. Cook about 4 to 5 minutes per side.
4   Put it together!
5   Add your favorite fixin like cheese, tomatoes, onions, or pickles.
6   Serve on buns or rolls.

Salmon with tarragon dill cream sauce

SERVES: 2

INGREDIENTS

Salmon Filets

• 1 1/2 lb. Salmon Filet

• 3/4-1 tsp. Dried Tarragon

• 3/4-1 tsp. Dried Dill Weed

• 1 tbsp. Duck Fat

• Salt and Pepper to Taste

Cream Sauce

• 2 tbsp. Butter

• 1/4 cup Heavy Cream

• 1/2 tsp. Dried Tarragon

• 1/2 tsp. Dried Dill Weed

• Salt and Pepper to Taste

DIRECTIONS

1. Slice the salmon in half to create 2 1/4 lb. filets. Season meat of fish with tarragon, dill weed, and salt and pepper. Turn around and season skin with salt and pepper only.

2. Heat 1 tbsp. duck fat in a ceramic cast-iron skillet over medium heat (or any

pan that will hold heat well). Once hot, add salmon skin side down.

3. Allow salmon to cook for 4-6 minutes while skinning crisps up. Once the skin is

crisp, reduce to low heat and flip salmon.

4. Cook salmon until the done-ness you want is achieved. Generally about 7-15

minutes over low heat.

Optional: If desired, cook on sides for 20-40 seconds to get darker edges.

5. Remove salmon from the pan and set it aside. Add butter and spices to the

pan and let brown. Once browned, add cream mix together.

6. Serve with broccoli or asparagus (or your favorite side dish) and be generous with cream sauce. Garnish with a small number of red pepper flakes.

Clam Loaf

SERVES: 1

INGREDIENTS

- 1 can clam, minced
- 1 or 2 eggs
- 1 pound. ground pork sausage
- 1 cup soda cracker crumbs
- Salt and pepper

DIRECTIONS

1 Drain clams, then mince.

2 Form all ingredients into a loaf and bake in a loaf pan for 40 minutes at 350 degrees F.

3 Serve hot or cold.

Clams Casino

SERVES: 6

INGREDIENTS

- 24 Cherrystone clams
- 2 tablespoons olive oil
- 1 tablespoon butter
- 1/2 cup finely minced onion
- 1/4 cup finely minced green bell pepper
- 2 cloves garlic, chopped
- 1 cup bread crumbs
- 4 slices crisply–fried bacon, crumbled
- 1/2 teaspoon oregano
- 2 tablespoons grated Parmesan cheese
- 1/4 cup very finely chopped parsley
- Paprika to taste
- Olive oil to taste

DIRECTIONS

1 Preheat oven to 450°F.
2 Wash and scrub clams well, discarding any that are open. Place on a baking sheet and bake until shells open, discarding any that do not open. Remove meat and chop. Discard half the shells.
3 Sauté onion, bell pepper, and garlic in oil and butter until soft. Remove from heat and cool. Add bread crumbs, bacon, oregano, Parmesan, and

reserved clams to onion mixture; mix well. Fill shells with clam mixture. Sprinkle with parsley and paprika; drizzle with olive oil. Bake for 7 minutes or until lightly browned. Remove from oven.

4   Serve hot.

Clams Italiano

SERVES: 2

INGREDIENTS

- dozen littleneck clams
- 1/4 cup dry white wine
- 1 cup bottled marinara sauce
- tablespoons chopped cilantro
- tablespoons chopped scallions

DIRECTIONS

1   Scrub clams well under cold running water.

2   Place in a microwave−safe dish with wine.

3   Microwave on high for 3 to 5 minutes until shells open. Discard any unopened clams.

4   Meanwhile, combine marinara, parsley, and scallions. Spoon over clams.

5   Microwave on medium−high for 2 minutes.

Clams Oregano Basilico

SERVES: 4

INGREDIENTS

- 36 Clams
- tablespoon Grated Romano cheese
- 2/3 tablespoon Dry white wine
- tablespoon Minced fresh Italian parsley
- Stuffing:
- 1/2 cup Fresh bread crumbs
- Juice of 1/2 Lemon (approx. 2 Tab)
- 1 tablespoon fresh basil
- 1 tablespoon Oregano
- 1 tablespoon Minced garlic

DIRECTIONS

1. Combine all stuffing ingredients by mixing with hands. Use more olive oil if the mixture seems too dry.
2. Preheat oven to 500 F. Shuck clams and replace meat on half–shells. Pack about 1 heaping tbs. stuffing on each. Bake in preheated oven for about 10 minutes.
3. Remove from oven and sprinkle each clam with a few drops of wine. Return to oven and bake 2 to 3 minutes more, or until lightly browned.

Grilled cod escabeche

SERVES: 4

INGREDIENTS

- cups Adobo Marinade
- ¾cup sliced pimento-stuffed Spanish green olives
- ¾cup finely chopped red onion
- ¾cup finely chopped red bell pepper
- 1 large jalapeno chile pepper, seeded
- tablespoons red wine vinegar
- 1 teaspoon sugar
- ¾teaspoon red pepper ßakes
- cod fillets (about 6 ounces each)
- 1 tablespoon olive oil
- ¾cup Orange-Cumin Rub

DIRECTIONS

1 Combine the marinade, olives, onion, bell pepper, jalapeno pepper, vinegar, sugar, and red pepper flakes in a small saucepan. Bring to a boil over high heat and boil for 1 minute. Remove from the heat and set aside.

2 Light a grill for direct medium-high heat, about 425¼F. Preheat a fish basket on the grill.

3 Coat the fish with olive oil, and then sprinkle the rub all over it.

4   Brush the grill grate and coat the grate and the hot fish basket generously with oil. Put the fillets in the basket and the basket on the grill, directly over the heat.

5   Cover and grill until the fish looks opaque on the surface, but is still filmy and moist in the center (an internal temperature of 130¼F), 2 to

6   minutes per side. Transfer the fillets to a large, shallow, nonreactive dish such as a 13-by-9-inch baking dish. Pour the marinade mixture over the fish and let cool to room temperature. Cover and refrigerate for at least 6 hours or up to 2 days. Return to room temperature before serving.

Buffalo CodQuesadilla

SERVES: 4

INGREDIENTS

- Salt and pepper to taste
- Monterey Jack cheese, shredded-1/2 cup
- Buffalo wingsauce, prepared-1 Tbsp
- Olive oil-2 Tbs
- 1 Alaskacod fillet-3 OZ
- Flour tortilla (8-inch)-1
- Tomatoes, diced (cut in very small pieces)-1/2 cup

DIRECTIONS

1 Season cod fillet by sprinkling with salt and pepper. Have an adult help you sauté the cod fillet in olive oil for 2 minutes.

2 Carefully turn and cook for another 2 to 3 minutes until fish is opaque throughout. (That means the flesh of the fish is no longer see-through.)

3 Remove from heat and when the cod is cool enough, take your fork and flake the meat. Refrigerate until needed.

4 Lay tortilla flat and build quesadilla on one half. Layer tortilla with cheese, tomatoes, the prepared cod, and buffalo wing sauce.

5 Fold in half and carefully lay on a hot, lightly oiled griddle.

6 Cook until the bottom is light brown. Carefully turn and cook until cheese is melted and the second side of the quesadilla is lightly browned.

7 Cut the tortilla into four triangles and enjoy!

MEDITERRANEAN PASTA

Viking Noodle Soup

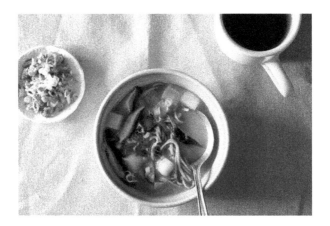

PREP TIME: 10 Minutes

COOKING TIME: 36 Minutes

SERVES 4

INGREDIENTS

- 2 tsp olive oil or 2 tsp vegetable oil
- 1/2 tsp salt
- 2 leeks, cleaned and chopped
- 1/4 tsp fresh ground black pepper
- 2 carrots, peeled and chopped
- 8 C. reduced-
- 1 garlic clove, minced
- chicken broth
- 1 stalk celery, chopped
- 6 oz. egg noodles, uncooked
- 3 -4 C. cooked turkey, shredded

- 1 C. frozen green pea
- 2 -3 bay leaves
- 2 tbsp fresh parsley leaves, chopped
- 2 tsp dried thyme

DIRECTIONS

1. In a large pan, heat the oil on medium heat, sauté the carrots, celery, leeks, and garlic for about 4 minutes.
2. Stir in the turkey, thyme, bay leaves, and black pepper.
3. Add the broth and bring it to a boil.
4. Reduce the heat to medium-low and simmer, covered partially for about 10 minutes.
5. Uncover and again bring to a boil, then stir in the noodles.
6. Simmer for about 10 minutes.
7. Stir in the peas and simmer for about 1 minute.
8. Remove everything from the heat and discard the bay leaves.
9. Stir in the parsley and serve.

NUTRITIONAL VALUES

Calories 536.3, Fat 12.8g, Cholesterol 115.7mg, Sodium 629.1mg, Carbohydrates 55.8g, Protein 51.1g

Egg noodle in Germany

PREP TIME: 10 Minutes

COOKING TIME: 15 Minutes

SERVES 6

INGREDIENTS

- kosher salt
- 3 tbsp flat-leaf parsley, chopped
- 1 (12 oz.) packages wide egg noodles
- fresh ground black pepper
- 4 -6 tbsp cold unsalted butter, cut into
- bits

DIRECTIONS

1. In a large pan of lightly salted boiling water, cook the egg noodles for about 5 minutes, stirring occasionally.

2. Drain well, reserving 1/4 C. of the cooking liquid.

3. In a medium skillet, add the reserved hot cooking liquid on low heat.

4. Slowly, add the butter, beating continuously till a creamy sauce forms.

5. Stir in the parsley, salt, and black pepper.

6. Add the noodles and toss to coat well.

7. Serve immediately.

NUTRITIONAL VALUES

Calories 287.4, Fat 10.2g, Cholesterol 68.2mg, Sodium 14.0mg, Carbohydrates 40.7g, Protein 8.2g

Italian Noodles with Croutons

PREP TIME: 5 Minutes

COOKING TIME: 20 Minutes

SERVES 4

INGREDIENTS

- 12 oz. egg noodles
- 1 pinch salt
- 1/2 C. unsalted butter
- 1/4 tsp pepper
- 2 slices white bread (day old is good),
- torn

DIRECTIONS

1. In a large pan of boiling water, prepare the egg noodles according to the package's directions.

2. Meanwhile for croutons in a small frying pan, melt the butter on medium heat and cook the bread pieces till lightly crispy.

3. Stir in the salt and black pepper and remove everything from the heat.

4. In a serving bowl, mix the noodles and croutons and serve

NUTRITIONAL VALUES

Calories 565.3, Fat 27.2g, Cholesterol 132.8mg, Sodium 145.0mg, Carbohydrates 67.3g, Protein 13.3g

Easy Homemade Egg

PREP TIME: 5 Minutes

COOKING TIME: 25 Minutes

SERVES 1

INGREDIENTS

- 6 eggs, beaten
- oil, for pan
- 1/2 C. water, room temperature
- 1/4 C. potato starch
- salt

DIRECTIONS

1. In a bowl, mix the potato starch and water.
2. Slowly, add the beaten eggs and salt, beating continuously till well combined.
3. Heat a lightly greased skillet on medium heat and add a thin layer of the egg mixture and cook till set.
4. Flip the side and immediately transfer onto a plate, uncooked side up.
5. Tightly roll it and cut everything into 1/4-inch circles.
6. Repeat with the remaining egg mixture.
7. These noodles can be used in any soup.

NUTRITIONAL VALUES

Calories 114.3, Fat 5.7g, Cholesterol 223.2mg, Sodium 90.3mg, Carbohydrates 7.0g, Protein 8.0g

Mexican Noodle Bake

PREP TIME: 20 Minutes

COOKING TIME: 90 Minutes

SERVES 4

INGREDIENTS

- 1 (8 oz.) packages wide egg noodles
- sauce
- 1 lb. lean ground beef
- 1/8 tsp pepper
- 6 green onions, sliced
- 1 (8 oz.) packages ricotta cheese
- 2 large garlic cloves, minced
- 1 C. sour cream
- 3/4 tsp salt, divided
- 1/2 C. shredded parmesan cheese
- 1 (26 oz.) jars tomato and basil pasta

DIRECTIONS

1. Set your oven to 350 degrees F before doing anything else and lightly grease a large baking dish.
2. Heat a large skillet on medium-high heat and cook the beef with green onions, garlic, and 1/2 tsp of the salt till the beef is browned completely.
3. Drain the excess grease from the skillet.
4. Stir in the pasta sauce and black pepper and reduce the heat.

5. Simmer, covered for about 20 minutes.

6. Meanwhile, cook the noodles according to the package's directions.

7. Drain well and transfer into a large bowl with 1 C. of the sour cream, ricotta, and remaining salt, then mix well.

8. Place half of the noodle mixture in the bottom of the prepared baking dish, followed by half of the beef mixture.

9. Repeat the layers and cook everything in the oven for about 25 minutes.

10. Sprinkle with Parmesan and cook everything in the oven for about 5 minutes more.

NUTRITIONAL VALUES

Calories 708.1, Fat 37.2g, Carbohydrates 47.6g, Protein 44.5g

VEGAN MAIN DISHES

Thai-Phoon Stir-Fry

SERVES: 4

INGREDIENTS

- 1 pound extra-firm tofu, drained and patted dry
- 2 tablespoons canola or grapeseed oil
- medium shallots halved lengthwise and cut into $\frac{1}{8}$-inch slices
- 2 garlic cloves, minced
- 2 teaspoons grated fresh ginger
- 3 ounces white mushroom caps, lightly rinsed, patted dry, and cut into $\frac{1}{2}$-inch slices
- 1 tablespoon creamy peanut butter
- 2 teaspoons light brown sugar
- 1 teaspoon Asian chili paste
- 2 tablespoons soy sauce
- 1 tablespoon mirin
- 1 (13.5-ounce) can unsweetened coconut milk
- 6 ounces chopped fresh spinach
- 1 tablespoon toasted sesame oil
- Freshly cooked rice or noodles, to serve
- 2 tablespoons finely chopped fresh Thai basil or cilantro
- 2 tablespoons crushed unsalted roasted peanuts
- 2 teaspoons minced crystallized ginger (optional)

DIRECTIONS

1. Cut the tofu into ½-inch dice and set aside. In a large skillet, heat 1 tablespoon of the oil over medium-high heat. Add the tofu and stir-fry until golden brown, about 7 minutes. Remove the tofu from the skillet and set it aside.

2. In the same skillet, heat the remaining 1 tablespoon oil over medium heat. Add shallots, garlic, ginger, and mushrooms and stir-fry until softened, about 4 minutes.

3. Stir in the peanut butter, sugar, chili paste, soy sauce, and mirin. Stir in the coconut milk and mix until well blended.

4. Add the fried tofu and the spinach and bring to a simmer.

5. Reduce the heat to medium-low and simmer, stirring occasionally, until the spinach is wilted and the flavors are well blended, 5 to 7 minutes.

6. Stir in the sesame oil and simmer for another minute. To serve, spoon the tofu mixture onto your choice of rice or noodles and top with coconut, basil, peanuts, and crystallized ginger if using. Serve immediately.

Chipotle-Painted Baked Tofu

SERVES: 4

INGREDIENTS

- 2 tablespoons soy sauce
- 2 canned chipotle chiles in adobo
- 1 tablespoon olive oil
- 1 pound extra-firm tofu, drained, cut into ½-inch thick slices, and pressed (see Light Vegetable Broth)

DIRECTIONS

1. Preheat the oven to 375°F. Lightly oil a 9 x 13-inch baking pan and set it aside.
2. In a food processor, combine the soy sauce, chipotles, and oil and process until blended. Scrape the chipotle mixture into a small bowl.
3. Brush the chipotle mixture onto both sides of the tofu slices and arrange them in a single layer in the prepared pan. Bake until hot, about 20 minutes. Serve immediately.

Grilled Tofu with Tamarind Glaze

SERVES: 4

INGREDIENTS

- 1 pound extra-firm tofu, drained and patted dry
- Salt and freshly ground black pepper
- 2 tablespoons olive oil
- 2 medium shallots, minced
- 2 garlic cloves, minced
- 2 ripe tomatoes, coarsely chopped
- 2 tablespoons ketchup
- ¼ cup water
- 2 tablespoons Dijon mustard
- 1 tablespoon dark brown sugar
- 2 tablespoons agave nectar
- 2 tablespoons tamarind concentrate
- 1 tablespoon dark molasses
- ½ teaspoon ground cayenne
- 1 tablespoon smoked paprika
- 1 tablespoon soy sauce

DIRECTIONS

Cut the tofu into 1-inch slices, season with salt and pepper to taste, and set aside in a shallow baking pan.

In a large saucepan, heat the oil over medium heat.

Add the shallots and garlic and sauté for 2 minutes. Add all the remaining ingredients, except for the tofu. Reduce the heat to low and simmer for 15 minutes. Transfer the mixture to a blender or food processor and blend until smooth. Return to the saucepan and cook 15 minutes longer, then set aside to cool. Pour the sauce over the tofu and refrigerate for at least 2 hours. Preheat a grill or broiler.

Grill the marinated tofu, turning once, to heat through, and brown nicely on both sides. While the tofu is grilling, reheat the marinade in a saucepan. Remove the tofu from the grill, brush each side with the tamarind sauce, and serve immediately.

Tofu Stuffed With Watercress And Tomatoes

SERVES: 4

INGREDIENTS

- 1 pound extra-firm tofu, drained, cut into ¾-inch slices, and pressed (see Light Vegetable Broth)
- Salt and freshly ground black pepper
- 1 small bunch watercress, tough stems removed and chopped
- 2 ripe plum tomatoes, chopped
- ½ cup minced green onions
- 2 tablespoons minced fresh parsley
- 2 tablespoons minced fresh basil
- 1 teaspoon minced garlic
- 2 tablespoons olive oil
- 1 tablespoon balsamic vinegar
- Pinch sugar
- ½ cup all-purpose flour
- ½ cup water
- 1½ cups dry unseasoned bread crumbs

DIRECTIONS

1. Cut a long deep pocket on the side of each slice of tofu and place the tofu on a baking sheet. Season with salt and pepper to taste and set aside.

2. In a large bowl, combine the watercress, tomatoes, green onions, parsley, basil, garlic, 2 tablespoons of the oil, vinegar, sugar, and salt and pepper to taste. Mix until well combined, then carefully stuff the mixture into the tofu pockets.

3. Place the flour in a shallow bowl. Pour the water into a separate shallow bowl. Place the bread crumbs on a large plate. Dredge the tofu in the flour, then carefully dip it in the water, and then dredge it in the bread crumbs, coating thoroughly.

4. In a large skillet, heat the remaining 2 tablespoons oil over medium heat. Add the stuffed tofu to the skillet and cook until golden brown, turning once, 4 to 5 minutes per side. Serve immediately.

Tofu with Pistachio-Pomegranate Sauce

SERVES: 4

INGREDIENTS

- 1 pound extra-firm tofu, drained, cut into ¼-inch slices, and pressed (see Light Vegetable Broth)
- Salt and freshly ground black pepper
- 2 tablespoons olive oil
- ½ cup pomegranate juice
- 1 tablespoon balsamic vinegar
- 1 tablespoon light brown sugar
- 2 green onions, minced
- ½ cup unsalted shelled pistachios, coarsely chopped
- Season the tofu with salt and pepper to taste.

DIRECTIONS

1. In a large skillet, heat the oil over medium heat. Add the tofu slices, in batches if necessary, and cook until lightly browned, about 4 minutes per side. Remove from skillet and set aside.
2. In the same skillet, add the pomegranate juice, vinegar, sugar, and green onions and simmer over medium heat, for 5 minutes. Add half of the pistachios and cook until sauce is slightly thickened about 5 minutes.

3. Return the fried tofu to the skillet and cook until hot, about 5 minutes, spooning the sauce over the tofu as it simmers. Serve immediately, sprinkled with the remaining pistachios.

Spice Island Tofu

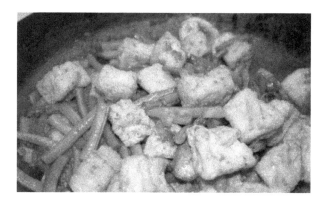

SERVES: 4

INGREDIENTS

- ½ cup cornstarch
- ½ teaspoon minced fresh thyme or ¼ teaspoon dried
- ½ teaspoon minced fresh marjoram or ¼ teaspoon dried
- ½ teaspoon salt
- ¼ teaspoon ground cayenne
- ¼ teaspoon sweet or smoked paprika
- ¼ teaspoon light brown sugar
- ⅛ teaspoon ground allspice
- 1 pound extra-firm tofu, drained and cut into ½-inch strips
- 2 tablespoons canola or grapeseed oil
- 1 medium red bell pepper, cut into ¼-inch strips
- 2 green onions, chopped
- 1 garlic cloves, minced

- 1 jalapeño, seeded and minced
- 2 ripe plum tomatoes, seeded and chopped
- 1 cup chopped fresh or canned pineapple
- 2 tablespoons soy sauce
- ¼ cup water
- 2 teaspoons fresh lime juice
- 1 tablespoon minced fresh parsley, for garnish

DIRECTIONS

1. In a shallow bowl, combine the cornstarch, thyme, marjoram, salt, cayenne, paprika, sugar, and allspice. Mix well. Dredge the tofu in the spice mixture, the coating on all sides. Preheat the oven to 250°F.

2. In a large skillet, heat 2 tablespoons of the oil over medium heat. Add the dredged tofu, in batches if necessary and cook until golden brown, about 4 minutes per side. Transfer the fried tofu to a heatproof platter and keep warm in the oven.

3. In the same skillet, heat the remaining 1 tablespoon oil over medium heat. Add the bell pepper, green onions, garlic, and jalapeño. Cover and cook, stirring occasionally, until tender, about 10 minutes.

4. Add the tomatoes, pineapple, soy sauce, water, and lime juice and simmer until the mixture is hot and the flavors have combined for about 5 minutes. Spoon the vegetable mixture over the fried tofu. Sprinkle with minced parsley and serve immediately.

Ginger Tofu with Citrus-Hoisin Sauce

SERVES: 4

INGREDIENTS

- 1 pound extra-firm tofu, drained, patted dry, and cut into ½-inch cubes
- 2 tablespoons soy sauce
- 2 tablespoons plus 1 teaspoon cornstarch
- 1 tablespoon plus 1 teaspoon canola or grapeseed oil
- 1 teaspoon toasted sesame oil
- 2 teaspoons grated fresh ginger
- green onions, minced
- ⅓ cup hoisin sauce
- ½ cup vegetable broth, homemade (see Light Vegetable Broth) or store-bought
- ¼ cup fresh orange juice
- 1½ tablespoons fresh lime juice
- 1½ tablespoons fresh lemon juice
- Salt and freshly ground black pepper

DIRECTIONS

1. Place the tofu in a shallow bowl.
2. Add the soy sauce and toss to coat, then sprinkle with 2 tablespoons of cornstarch and toss to coat.

3. In a large skillet, heat 1 tablespoon of the canola oil over medium heat. Add the tofu and cook until golden brown, turning occasionally, about 10 minutes. Remove the tofu from the pan and set it aside.

4. In the same skillet, heat the remaining 1 teaspoon canola oil and the sesame oil over medium heat. Add the ginger and green onions and cook until fragrant, about 1 minute. Stir in the hoisin sauce, broth, and orange juice and bring to a simmer.

5. Cook until the liquid is reduced slightly and the flavors have a chance to meld for about 3 minutes.

6. In a small bowl, combine the remaining 1 teaspoon cornstarch with the lime juice and lemon juice and add to the sauce, stirring to thicken slightly. Season with salt and pepper to taste.

7. Return the fried tofu to the skillet and cook until coated with the sauce and heated through. Serve immediately.

Tofu with Lemongrass And Snow Peas

SERVES: 4

INGREDIENTS

- 2 tablespoons canola or grapeseed oil
- 1 medium red onion, halved and thinly sliced
- 2 garlic cloves, minced
- 1 teaspoon grated fresh ginger
- 1 pound extra-firm tofu, drained and cut into ½-inch dice
- 2 tablespoons soy sauce
- 1 tablespoon mirin or sake
- 1 teaspoon sugar
- ½ teaspoon crushed red pepper
- 4 ounces snow peas, trimmed
- 1 tablespoon minced lemongrass or zest of 1 lemon
- 2 tablespoons coarsely ground unsalted roasted peanuts, for garnish

DIRECTIONS

1. In a large skillet or wok, heat the oil over medium-high heat. Add the onion, garlic, and ginger and stir-fry for 2 minutes.
2. Add the tofu and cook until golden brown, about 7 minutes.
3. Stir in the soy sauce, mirin, sugar, and crushed red pepper.
4. Add the snow peas and lemongrass and stir-fry until the snow peas are crisp-tender and the flavors are well blended for about 3 minutes.
5. Garnish with peanuts and serve immediately.

Double-Sesame Tofu with Tahini Sauce

SERVES: 4

INGREDIENTS

- ½ cup tahini (sesame paste)
- 2 tablespoons fresh lemon juice
- 2 tablespoons soy sauce
- 2 tablespoons water
- ¼ cup white sesame seeds
- ¼ cup black sesame seeds
- ½ cup cornstarch
- 1 pound extra-firm tofu, drained, patted dry, and cut into ½-inch strips
- Salt and freshly ground black pepper
- 2 tablespoons canola or grapeseed oil

DIRECTIONS

1. In a small bowl, combine the tahini, lemon juice, soy sauce, and water, stirring to blend well. Set aside.
2. In a shallow bowl, combine the white and black sesame seeds and cornstarch, stirring to blend. Season the tofu with salt and pepper to taste. Set aside.

3. In a large skillet, heat the oil over medium heat. Dredge the tofu in the sesame seed mixture until well coated, then add to the hot skillet and cook until browned and crispy all over, turning as needed, 3 to 4 minutes per side. Be careful not to burn the seeds.

4. Drizzle with tahini sauce and serve immediately.

Tofu And Edamame Stew

SERVES: 4

INGREDIENTS

- 2 tablespoons olive oil
- 1 medium yellow onion, chopped
- ½ cup chopped celery
- 2 garlic cloves, minced
- 2 medium Yukon Gold potatoes, peeled and cut into ½-inch dice
- 1 cup shelled fresh or frozen edamame
- 2 cups peeled and diced zucchini
- ½ cup frozen baby peas
- 1 teaspoon dried savory
- ½ teaspoon crumbled dried sage
- ⅛ teaspoon ground cayenne
- 1½ cups vegetable broth, homemade (see Light Vegetable Broth) or store-bought Salt and freshly ground black pepper
- 1 pound extra-firm tofu, drained, patted dry, and cut into ½-inch dice
- 2 tablespoons minced fresh parsley

DIRECTIONS

1   In a large saucepan, heat 1 tablespoon of the oil over medium heat. Add the onion, celery, and garlic. Cover and cook until softened, about 10 minutes. Stir in the potatoes, edamame, zucchini, peas, savory, sage, and cayenne.

2   Add the broth and bring to a boil. Reduce heat to low and season with salt and pepper to taste. Cover and simmer until the vegetables are tender and the flavors are blended for about 40 minutes.

3   In a large skillet, heat the remaining 1 tablespoon oil over medium-high heat. Add the tofu and cook until golden brown, about 7 minutes. Season with salt and pepper to taste and set aside. About 10 minutes before the stew is finished cooking, add the fried tofu and parsley. Taste, adjusting seasonings if necessary, and serve immediately.

COOKING CONVERSION CHART

TEMPERATURE		WEIGHT	
FAHRENHEIT	**CELSIUS**	**IMPERIAL**	**METRIC**
100 °F	37 °C	1/2 oz	15 g
150 °F	65 °C	1 oz	29 g
200 °F	93 °C	2 oz	57 g
250 °F	121 °C	3 oz	85 g
300 °F	150 °C	4 oz	113 g
325 °F	160 °C	5 oz	141 g
350 °F	180 °C	6 oz	170 g
375 °F	190 °C	8 oz	227 g
400 °F	200 °C	10 oz	283 g
425 °F	220 °C	12 oz	340 g
450 °F	230 °C	13 oz	369 g
500 °F	260 °C	14 oz	397 g
525 °F	270 °C	15 oz	425 g
550 °F	288 °C	1 lb	453 g

MEASUREMENT			
CUP	ONCES	MILLILITERS	TABLESPOON
1/16 cup	1/2 oz	15 ml	1
1/8 cup	1 oz	30 ml	3
1/4 cup	2 oz	59 ml	4
1/3 cup	2.5 oz	79 ml	5.5
3/8 cup	3 oz	90 ml	6
1/2 cup	4 oz	118 ml	8
2/3 cup	5 oz	158 ml	11
3/4 cup	6 oz	177 ml	12
1 cup	8 oz	240 ml	16
2 cup	16 oz	480 ml	32
4 cup	32 oz	960 ml	64
5 cup	40 oz	1180 ml	80
6 cup	48 oz	1420 ml	96
8 cup	64 oz	1895 ml	128

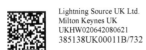

9 781802 353976